Table of Contents

What is The Vertical Diet?

The Vertical Diet is a diet that is based on whole foods that are high in nutrients. It is promoted through claims to optimise gut-health and improve performance. A "horizontal" diet would be described as one that emphasises a wide variety of foods. The Vertical Diet, therefore, focuses on a limited number of foods that Stan Efferding has chosen for specific reasons.

One of the pieces of reasoning behind this is that it is hypothesised that limiting the variety can help the body become more efficient at digesting the foods that are consumed. This would allow for better absorption of nutrients, while also making it easier to eat more total food volume across the day.

According to Efferding, this limited variety and improved digestive efficiency should improve muscle growth, recovery, gut health, and metabolism. The vertical component of the diet includes red meat and white rice. These are designed to make up the majority of the calories.

Red meat is chosen because it is a quality protein source that is also higher in iron, B vitamins and zinc than other options. White rice is chosen as the main carbohydrate source because it is easy to consume a lot of carbohydrates through and it doesn't take long to digest. This makes it easier for heavier strength athletes to consume more carbohydrates and calories.

Within the horizontal component of the diet, there is more variety as these foods are chosen to meet micronutrient needs. They are specifically nutrient-dense; however, the goal is to consume them in an appropriate amount and no more than that. They are designed to reach the optimal targets for micronutrient needs and no more. Adding more micronutrients than this level typically does not provide any additional benefit, so the preference is to focus the majority of the diet on the vertical component once these needs are met.

The foods chosen are generally low-FODMAP as well. They are designed to limit gas build-up and the bloating or other gastrointestinal issues related to that.

Why is it called the Vertical Diet?

The Vertical Diet is named as such because it's pictured graphically as an upside-down T. "Imagine that the base of the T is represented by foods rich in vitamins and minerals, and the vertical portion of the T is made up of red meat and white rice," notes Susie. Essentially, the basis of the diet is that it allows people to consume larger amounts of food without getting full, resulting in higher calorie consumption and more energy. It's also very heavily focussed on meat, so isn't suitable for vegetarians or vegans.

How to follow the Vertical Diet

The Vertical Diet has several components, all of which are meant to maximize muscle gain. While designed to be high in carbs, the diet can also be customized to meet a variety of eating patterns, including low-carb diets, intermittent fasting, and the paleo diet.

Primary foods

Red meat and white rice comprise the bulk of the Vertical Diet.

According to the diet's advocates, white rice is the primary carb source because it's easy to digest, especially in large quantities. This is particularly important for serious athletes with very high calorie needs.

Red meat is preferred over poultry or fish due to its nutrient density and concentration of iron, B vitamins, zinc, and cholesterol, which the diet claims are important for muscle growth and testosterone production.

However, as you can't meet all your micronutrient needs with these two foods, the diet includes a limited amount of nutrient-rich, easily digestible foods, such as eggs, yogurt, spinach, and salmon.

Restrictions

All foods that aren't easily digestible are discouraged.

These include vegetables that may cause bloating and gas, such as broccoli and cauliflower, which are high in FODMAPs, as well as onion and garlic.

Legumes, brown rice, and other grains are also curbed because they contain lectins and phytic acid, which may limit your absorption of certain nutrients (1Trusted Source, 2Trusted Source).

However, small amounts of legumes and oats are allowed as long as they're sprouted or soaked to make them easier to digest.

Steps to follow

When starting out, you calculate your basal metabolic rate (BMR), or the number of calories your body needs to function while at rest. You then add calories based on your training regimen. Bodybuilders should aim for a calorie surplus to gain muscle weight. As your body adjusts to the diet and starts to feel hungry between meals, you're supposed to "go vertical" by adding more calories. This process is meant to support greater muscle gains, quicker recovery, and more intense or frequent training sessions.

The exact number of additional calories is based on training needs and involves either increasing your portions of rice and meat or eating an additional meal during the day. Once you start feeling hungry between meals again, you repeat this process until you've reached your goal weight or goal muscle mass.

What Foods You Can Eat on the Vertical Diet

The two most commonly eaten foods on this diet are red meat and white rice. White rice because it's incredibly easy and fast to digest (think: quick energy). Red meat for its iron, zinc, selenium, and B vitamins, as well as its muscle-building potential. (Low-FODMAP foods also are addressed. Read more about the what foods you can and can't eat on a low-FODMAP diet.)

- Red meat, preferably grass-fed bison and beef. Skip pre-ground beef as its usually made from scraps, according to Vertical Diet advocates.
- Hormone-free chicken
- Beef tallow and other "unprocessed" fats
- Line-caught salmon
- Eggs
- Full-fat dairy
- Low-gas vegetables, as defined by FODMAP, such as spinach, cucumbers, and bell peppers
- All fruits, with a focus on low-FODMAP ones
- Sprouted or soaked legumes and oats, but only in small quantities

What Foods You Can't Eat on the Vertical Diet

- Brown rice and other grains
- Processed vegetable oils (which is essentially any vegetable oil)
- Legumes, including soy
- Onions and garlic
- Coffee
- Added sugar and sugar alcohols

- High-FODMAP vegetables, also referred to as high-raffinose or gas-causing vegetables

Pros of The Vertical Diet:

There is no doubt that The Vertical Diet can be an option to help fuel elite performance. There are a lot of people taking their performance to the next level while utilising the diet, so it is worthwhile looking at the positives.

Less Bloating

Due to the emphasis on low-FODMAP foods and avoiding any foods that are difficult to digest, The Vertical Diet can reduce bloating, constipation and diarrhoea in a lot of individuals. This alone can improve quality of life and make people feel better.

Easier Way to Eat More Food

Due to the focus on easily digestible foods, it allows people to eat more total food. Generally, when strength athletes focus on high quality, nutrient-dense foods, they struggle to consume enough calories to maintain or gain weight. This can harm strength performance, which in turn limits their potential as an athlete.

Emphasising the foods in The Vertical Diet can overcome this barrier. The meal plans are also laid out in a way that makes it easier to consume large amounts of food. There is also a strategic way laid out to increase food intake.

Can Be an Easy Way to Adjust Intake Since It Is So Consistent

The diet can be great from the perspective of keeping it simple. When there is a lot of variety, it can be harder to consistently get an appropriate range of calories and macros for your specific goals, unless you are tracking your intake.

With The Vertical Diet, you will generally have pretty much the same 4-5 meals per day every day. If you wanted to gain size but weren't in a calorie surplus, you have the option to either make the meals larger or add an additional meal.

Vice-versa, if somebody wanted to be in a calorie deficit, they could do the opposite. This makes it really easy to adjust your calories based on your needs.

Good Focus on Micronutrients and Performance

Sometimes concepts such as flexible dieting can be taken too far and completely underrate the importance of micronutrients. The Vertical Diet has an emphasis on ensuring all micronutrient needs are met, which can have carryover effects for performance.

While going above these levels might not have additional benefits, avoiding deficiencies or inadequacies is important. Using iron as one example of this, if somebody was deficient in iron, they would feel fatigued and their training wouldn't be as effective.

Performance is also optimised from a macronutrient standpoint too. The diet can be laid out in a way that meets appropriate ranges for protein, fats and carbs, while also distributing protein across the day.

Focus on Non-Dietary Details

Not only is there a focus on the dietary aspects, but there is also a focus on lifestyle overall. In the book, there is a lot of time dedicated to things such as sleep, short walks and regular blood tests.

There is so much evidence that getting sufficient good quality sleep will help performance, but it is often overlooked. Short walks directly after a meal can help reduce blood glucose levels (mostly only relevant for people at risk of T2DM, but it can be particularly important for people at very high BMI's in general). Getting regular comprehensive blood tests can help identify any issues early on that can be addressed, which can help improve health and performance.

Cons of The Vertical Diet:

Red Meat Is Expensive

Red meat is more expensive than other protein sources. While red meat isn't the only protein source on the diet, it is the main form that is emphasised. The reason red meat is chosen over white meat such as chicken is that it is slightly higher in nutrients.

Switching some of the red meat for white meat really would have no negatives though. After reaching certain targets for micronutrients such as iron, zinc and B vitamins, there is no noticeable benefit for going higher. At the food volumes consumed, there is no doubt those targets would be met even if white meat was the preferential choice. This switch alone can make the diet a lot cheaper without sacrificing anything from a performance perspective.

Caution Regarding Red Meat and Health

While there have been certain recent guidelines suggesting that we do not need to reduce our current intake of red meat for health purposes, I'm of the opinion that it would be wise to be mildly cautious of going anywhere near as high what the vertical diet proposes.

The vast majority of organisations have guidelines that recommend limiting red meat intake, with a particular emphasis on the linkage with bowel cancer.

There is a reason they have those guidelines in place and it takes a lot of confidence (or audacity) in your own research skills to believe that your interpretation of the evidence is better than these organisations.

There is a wealth of research out on this topic, but due to the variables involved it is hard to make a clear conclusion, which is part of why I'm choosing not to discuss the research here as I think that should be a separate article by itself. Healthy user bias can mask what is really going on. For example, people who eat red meat are also more likely to partake in behaviours with negative effects on health, whereas those who follow plant-based diets tend to do the opposite.

With that being said, while I believe I am more comfortable with higher intakes of red meat than most dietitians, I still stand in the camp of caution and wouldn't take red meat intake to an extreme.

Staying on a Low-Fodmap Diet Indefinitely Isn't Ideal for Gut-Health

While The Vertical Diet isn't specifically a low-FODMAP diet, it comes very close. It eliminates most prominent gas-producing foods, which often overlap with high-FODMAP foods.

Since a lot of high-FODMAP foods are also great prebiotics, it appears as though staying low-FODMAP reduces microbial diversity in the gut. It also reduces the amount of Bifidobacterium and Lactobacillus which are associated with positive health outcomes.

Variety Can Be Beneficial for Gut Health

While The Vertical Diet reduces IBS type symptoms off the bat, claiming it optimises gut-health is a stretch. There is research indicating that consuming >30 plant-based foods is linked with greater microbial diversity and associated with more health-promoting groups of bacteria when compared to <10 per week.

Gut health is complex, and it is hard to make bold claims, but variety appears to be beneficial. Limiting to only a small number of foods like The Vertical Diet recommends could have negative effects due to this.

Needlessly Restrictive

In addition to a lot of the pitfalls associated with the restriction, there really isn't much evidence to support the idea that digestion is improved by limiting to the same foods over and over again. You can get the same results without restricting to this level.

How long should you be on the Vertical Diet for?

"The Vertical Diet is more of a short-term, performance-focused diet, not necessarily a lifestyle change," says Susie. "It's important to note that the main reason people follow it is to support muscle growth and digestion in bodybuilders." Bodybuilders, weightlifters, and athletes see the diet as a way to increase calorie consumption, but maintain gut health, on a temporary basis.

Is the Vertical Diet dangerous?

"Generally speaking, the Vertical Diet is highly restrictive and doesn't allow for enough of the nutrients your body needs to stay healthy," says Susie. "The diet places a focus on red meat as the primary source of your protein, but high red meat consumption is linked to heart disease, some cancers, kidney problems and digestive issues." Overall, a more balanced and nutrient-rich diet is a healthier option for the average gym-goer.

Recipes

Sweet Potato and Kale Scrambled Eggs

Recipe Summary

prep: 10 mins

cook: 10 mins

total: 20 mins

Servings: 2

Yield: 2 servings

Ingredients

  1 ½ cups egg whites

  2 large eggs

1 dash hot sauce (such as Tabasco®), or to taste

ground black pepper to taste

1 tablespoon coconut oil

½ cup cubed cooked sweet potato

½ cup torn kale leaves

½ cup salsa

Directions

Instructions

Step 1

Whisk egg whites and eggs together in a bowl; add hot sauce and pepper.

Step 2

Heat coconut oil in a skillet over medium heat. Add sweet potato and kale; cook and stir until kale is wilted, about 5 minutes.

Step 3

Stir egg mixture into sweet potato mixture; cook, stirring constantly, until egg is cooked and set, about 5 minutes. Transfer egg mixture to serving plates and top with salsa.

Nutrition Facts

Per Serving:

290 calories; protein 28.8g; carbohydrates 18.1g; fat 12.1g; cholesterol 186mg; sodium 799.7mg.

Spicy Potatoes and Scrambled Eggs
Recipe Summary

prep: 10 mins

cook: 15 mins

total: 25 mins

Servings: 4

Yield: 3 to 4 servings

Ingredients

  2 potatoes, scrubbed

  4 tablespoons vegetable oil, divided

  3 eggs

  salt and pepper to taste

  ½ teaspoon ground cumin

½ teaspoon ground coriander

½ teaspoon turmeric powder

½ teaspoon chili powder

½ teaspoon salt

Directions

Instructions

Step 1

Poke potatoes with a fork so that their skins are pierced. Microwave potatoes on high until cooked inside. When potatoes are fully cooked, peel potatoes and cut potatoes to 1/8 size or to your liking. Set potatoes aside.

Step 2

Add 2 tablespoons oil to skillet and scramble 3 eggs. Add salt and pepper to taste. Keep warm until potatoes are ready.

Step 3

In another skillet, heat 2 tablespoons oil until hot. Then add salt, cumin, coriander and turmeric powder. Put in chili powder if you want it really spicy. Add potatoes and cook until potatoes are crispy and brown. Spicy potatoes and scrambled eggs are now ready to serve!

Nutrition Facts

Per Serving:

209 calories; protein 5.5g; carbohydrates 8.2g; fat 17.5g; cholesterol 139.5mg; sodium 350.5mg.

Loaded Cauliflower

Recipe Summary

prep: 10 mins

cook: 45 mins

total: 55 mins

Servings: 4

Yield: 4 servings

Ingredients

1 head cauliflower

½ cup sour cream

½ cup shredded Cheddar cheese

1 teaspoon dry ranch salad dressing mix (such as Hidden Valley Ranch®)

½ teaspoon onion powder

½ teaspoon garlic powder

1 tablespoon butter, cut into small pieces, or more to taste

Directions

Instructions

Step 1

Preheat oven to 350 degrees F (175 degrees C).

Step 2

Place a steamer insert into a saucepan and fill with water to just below the bottom of the steamer. Bring water to a boil. Add cauliflower, cover, and steam until very tender, 15 to 20 minutes. Transfer cauliflower to a bowl, mash, and strain excess water.

Step 3

Mix cauliflower, sour cream, Cheddar cheese, ranch dressing mix, onion powder, and garlic powder together in a 9-inch baking dish; top with butter.

Step 4

Bake in the preheated oven until bubbling, 30 to 45 minutes.

Nutrition Facts

Per Serving:

196 calories; protein 8.2g; carbohydrates 9.8g; fat 14.8g; cholesterol 38.4mg; sodium 226.9mg.

Waffle House® Breakfast Wannabe

Recipe Summary

prep: 10 mins

cook: 23 mins

total: 33 mins

Servings: 2

Yield: 2 servings

Ingredients

6 slices bacon

4 links turkey sausage, or more to taste

4 eggs

¼ cup shredded Italian 3-cheese blend

2 slices jalapeno pepper, minced

2 tablespoons vegetable oil, divided

1 (16 ounce) package frozen hash brown potatoes, thawed

½ cup salsa

Directions

Instructions

Step 1

Place bacon and sausage in a large skillet and cook over medium-high heat, turning occasionally, until evenly browned, about 10 minutes. Drain bacon slices and sausage on paper towels; crumble bacon and dice sausage.

Step 2

Whisk eggs, 3-cheese blend, and jalapeno pepper together in a bowl; add sausage.

Step 3

Heat 1 tablespoon oil in a skillet over medium heat; cook and stir egg mixture until cooked through and scrambled, 3 to 5 minutes.

Step 4

Heat 1 tablespoon oil in a large skillet over medium-high heat; cook and stir hash brown potatoes until cooked through and browned, about 10 minutes.

Step 5

Spoon scrambled eggs onto a plate and top with salsa and bacon. Serve potatoes alongside eggs.

Nutrition Facts

Per Serving:

902 calories; protein 60.7g; carbohydrates 45.7g; fat 67.2g; cholesterol 533.5mg; sodium 2609.7mg.

Mongolian Beef and Spring Onions

Recipe Summary

prep: 12 mins

cook: 8 mins

additional: 10 mins

total: 30 mins

Servings: 4

Yield: 4 servings

Ingredients

2 teaspoons vegetable oil

1 tablespoon finely chopped garlic

½ teaspoon grated fresh ginger root

½ cup soy sauce

½ cup water

⅔ cup dark brown sugar

1 pound beef flank steak, sliced 1/4 inch thick on the diagonal

¼ cup cornstarch

1 cup vegetable oil for frying

2 bunches green onions, cut in 2-inch lengths

Directions

Instructions

Step 1

Heat 2 teaspoons of vegetable oil in a saucepan over medium heat, and cook and stir the garlic and ginger until they release their fragrance, about 30 seconds. Pour in the soy sauce, water, and brown sugar. Raise the heat to medium-high, and stir 4 minutes, until the sugar has dissolved and the sauce boils and slightly thickens. Remove sauce from the heat, and set aside.

Step 2

Place the sliced beef into a bowl, and stir the cornstarch into the beef, coating it thoroughly. Allow the beef and cornstarch to sit until most of the juices from the meat have been absorbed by the cornstarch, about 10 minutes.

Step 3

Heat the vegetable oil in a deep-sided skillet or wok to 375 degrees F (190 degrees C).

Step 4

Shake excess cornstarch from the beef slices, and drop them into the hot oil, a few at a time. Stir briefly, and fry until the edges become crisp and start to brown, about 2 minutes. Remove the beef from the oil with a large slotted spoon, and allow to drain on paper towels to remove excess oil.

Step 5

Pour the oil out of the skillet or wok, and return the pan to medium heat. Return the beef slices to the pan, stir briefly, and pour in the reserved sauce. Stir once or twice to combine, and add the green onions. Bring the mixture to a boil, and cook until the onions have softened and turned bright green, about 2 minutes.

Nutrition Facts

Per Serving:

391 calories; protein 18g; carbohydrates 54.7g; fat 12.1g; cholesterol 27.2mg; sodium 1861.8mg.

Recipe Summary

prep: 10 mins

cook: 15 mins

total: 25 mins

Servings: 6

Yield: 6 servings

Ingredients

6 tablespoons butter

2 cloves garlic, minced

1 ½ tablespoons Cajun seasoning

1 teaspoon salt

1 teaspoon ground black pepper

1 pound raw shrimp, peeled and deveined

1 (12 ounce) package dry fettuccine pasta

⅓ cup all-purpose flour

2 cups milk

1 cup heavy whipping cream

1 tablespoon lemon juice

½ tablespoon soy sauce

Directions

Instructions

Step 1

Bring a pot of lightly salted water to a boil.

Step 2

Melt butter in a large skillet over medium-high heat. Saute garlic until fragrant, about 1 minute. Add Cajun seasoning, salt, and pepper. Add shrimp and cook for 1 to 1 1/2 minutes. Turn shrimp over and cook, about 1 to 1 1/2 minute more. Transfer to a bowl and cover with aluminum foil to keep warm, leaving the butter in the skillet.

Step 3

Place pasta in the boiling water; cook until tender yet firm to the bite, 8 to 10 minutes.

Step 4

Add flour to the butter in the skillet; cook for 30 seconds. Add milk, cream, lemon juice, and soy sauce. Reduce heat to medium-low. Cook and stir until flavors blend, about 5 minutes. Add the shrimp and cook until well coated and opaque, about 5 minutes more.

Step 5

Spoon the shrimp and sauce on top of the cooked pasta.

Cook's Notes:

For a thicker sauce reverse the amounts of heavy cream and milk. You can also add sliced mushrooms and/or 1/2 cup sour cream.

Nutrition Facts

Per Serving:

575 calories; protein 24.6g; carbohydrates 53.2g; fat 29.9g; cholesterol 206.4mg; sodium 1084mg.

Falafel Pita Sandwich with Tahini Sauce

Recipe Summary

prep: 20 mins

cook: 10 mins

total: 30 mins

Servings: 6

Yield: 6 sandwiches

Ingredients

12 frozen falafel

¼ cup tahini

¼ cup water

2 tablespoons lemon juice

2 cloves garlic, minced

¼ teaspoon ground paprika

6 whole wheat pitas

1 head lettuce, shredded

1 tomato, cut into thin wedges

½ cucumber, peeled and sliced

1 low-sodium dill pickle, sliced

¼ small red onion, thinly sliced

3 teaspoons harissa, or to taste (Optional)

Directions

Instructions

Step 1

Preheat the oven to 450 degrees F (230 degrees C). Place falafel on a baking sheet.

Step 2

Bake in the preheated oven until heated through, 8 to 10 minutes.

Step 3

While falafel bake, whisk tahini, water, lemon juice, garlic, and paprika together in a bowl.

Step 4

Cut about 1 inch from the top of each pita to form a pocket. Add 2 falafel to each pita with equal amounts lettuce, tomato, cucumber, pickle, and red onion. Drizzle each with about 1 tablespoon tahini sauce and some harissa.

Cook's Note:

You can use any hot sauce you like in place of harissa.

Nutrition Facts

Per Serving:

361 calories; protein 12.6g; carbohydrates 53.4g; fat 12.7g; sodium 576.4mg.

Recipe Summary

Servings: 24

Yield: 24 squares

Ingredients

¼ cup butter

4 cups miniature marshmallows

5 cups crisp rice cereal

Directions

Instructions

Step 1

Melt butter in large sauce pan over low heat. Add marshmallows and stir until melted and well-blended. Cook 2 minutes longer, stirring constantly. Remove from heat.

Step 2

Add cereal. Stir until well coated.

Step 3

Using buttered spatula or waxed paper, press mixture evenly and firmly in buttered 13 x 9 inch pan. Cut into 2 x 2 inch squares when cool.

Nutrition Facts

Per Serving:

65 calories; protein 0.6g; carbohydrates 11.8g; fat 2g; cholesterol 5.1mg; sodium 64.8mg.

Salsa Chicken

Recipe Summary

prep: 5 mins

cook: 40 mins

total: 45 mins

Servings: 4

Yield: 4 servings

Ingredients

4 skinless, boneless chicken breast halves

4 teaspoons taco seasoning mix

1 cup salsa

1 cup shredded Cheddar cheese

2 tablespoons sour cream (Optional)

Directions

Instructions

Step 1

Preheat oven to 375 degrees F (190 degrees C)

Step 2

Place chicken breasts in a lightly greased 9x13 inch baking dish. Sprinkle taco seasoning on both sides of chicken breasts, and pour salsa over all.

Step 3

Bake at 375 degrees F (190 degrees C) for 25 to 35 minutes, or until chicken is tender and juicy and its juices run clear.

Step 4

Sprinkle chicken evenly with cheese, and continue baking for an additional 3 to 5 minutes, or until cheese is melted and bubbly. Top with sour cream if desired, and serve.

Nutrition Facts

Per Serving:

287 calories; protein 35.5g; carbohydrates 6.8g; fat 12.4g; cholesterol 101.3mg; sodium 863.1mg.

Chinese Pepper Steak

Recipe Summary

prep: 15 mins

cook: 15 mins

total: 30 mins

Servings: 4

Yield: 4 servings

Ingredients

1 pound beef top sirloin steak

¼ cup soy sauce

2 tablespoons white sugar

2 tablespoons cornstarch

½ teaspoon ground ginger

3 tablespoons vegetable oil, divided

1 red onion, cut into 1-inch squares

1 green bell pepper, cut into 1-inch squares

2 tomatoes, cut into wedges

Directions

Instructions

Step 1

Slice the steak into 1/2-inch thick slices across the grain.

Step 2

Whisk together soy sauce, sugar, cornstarch, and ginger in a bowl until the sugar has dissolved and the mixture is smooth. Place the steak slices into the marinade, and stir until well-coated.

Step 3

Heat 1 tablespoon of vegetable oil in a wok or large skillet over medium-high heat, and place 1/3 of the steak strips into the hot oil. Cook and stir until the beef is well-browned, about 3 minutes, and remove the beef from the wok to a bowl. Repeat twice more, with the remaining beef, and set the cooked beef aside.

Step 4

Return all the cooked beef to the hot wok, and stir in the onion. Toss the beef and onion together until the onion begins to soften, about 2 minutes, then stir in the green pepper. Cook and stir the mixture until the pepper has turned bright green and started to become tender, about 2 minutes, then add the tomatoes, stir everything together, and serve.

Nutrition Facts

Per Serving:

312 calories; protein 26.1g; carbohydrates 17g; fat 15.4g; cholesterol 69.2mg; sodium 972.4mg.

Salsa Chicken Burrito Filling

Recipe Summary

prep: 5 mins

cook: 30 mins

total: 35 mins

Servings: 4

Yield: 4 servings

Ingredients

2 skinless, boneless chicken breast halves

1 (4 ounce) can tomato sauce

¼ cup salsa

1 (1.25 ounce) package taco seasoning mix

1 teaspoon ground cumin

2 cloves garlic, minced

1 teaspoon chili powder

hot sauce to taste

Directions

Instructions

Step 1

Place chicken breasts and tomato sauce in a medium saucepan over medium high heat. Bring to a boil, then add the salsa, seasoning, cumin, garlic and chili powder. Let simmer for 15 minutes.

Step 2

With a fork, start pulling the chicken meat apart into thin strings. Keep cooking pulled chicken meat and sauce, covered, for another 5 to 10 minutes. Add hot sauce to taste and stir together (Note: You may need to add a bit of water if the mixture is cooked too high and gets too thick.)

Nutrition Facts

Per Serving:

107 calories; protein 12.3g; carbohydrates 9.6g; fat 1.5g; cholesterol 30.4mg; sodium 923.4mg.

Creamy Cajun Shrimp Pasta

Recipe Summary

prep: 10 mins

cook: 10 mins

total: 20 mins

Servings: 4

Yield: 4 servings

Ingredients

1 (8 ounce) package angel hair pasta

¼ cup butter

1 pound shrimp, peeled and deveined

1 clove garlic, minced

¼ cup all-purpose flour

2 tablespoons Cajun seasoning

2 cups milk

¼ teaspoon salt

1 tablespoon lemon juice

Directions

Instructions

Step 1

Bring a large pot of lightly salted water to a boil. Add pasta and cook for 4 minutes or until al dente; drain.

Step 2

Melt butter in a large heavy skillet over medium heat. Saute shrimp for 1 minute on each side. Stir in garlic, and cook for 1 minute. Remove shrimp with a slotted spoon; set aside. Stir in flour and Cajun seasoning. Cook, stirring for 5 minutes. Gradually whisk in milk, then cook until thickened. Remove from heat, and season with salt and lemon juice. Return shrimp to sauce, and spoon over cooked pasta.

Nutrition Facts

Per Serving:

483 calories; protein 34.4g; carbohydrates 46g; fat 17.6g; cholesterol 212.8mg; sodium 1271.5mg.

Recipe Summary

prep: 15 mins

cook: 6 mins

total: 21 mins

Servings: 4

Yield: 2 cups stir-fry

Ingredients

- 2 ½ tablespoons dark sesame oil, divided

- 6 ounces shiitake mushroom caps, sliced

- 4 cups thinly sliced napa cabbage

- 1 tablespoon reduced-sodium soy sauce

- ¼ teaspoon freshly ground black pepper

- ¼ cup cilantro leaves

- 2 tablespoons toasted sesame seeds

Directions

Instructions

Step 1

Heat a large skillet over high heat. Add 2 tablespoons sesame oil; swirl to coat. Saute mushrooms until browned, about 4 minutes. Add cabbage; saute for 2 minutes.

Step 2

Remove skillet from heat. Mix in 1 1/2 teaspoon sesame oil, soy sauce, and black pepper until well combined. Top with cilantro and sesame seeds.

Nutrition Facts

Per Serving:

133 calories; protein 2.9g; carbohydrates 6.4g; fat 10.9g; sodium 150.9mg.

Latin-Inspired Spicy Cream Chicken Stew

Recipe Summary

prep: 10 mins

cook: 8 hrs 15 mins

total: 8 hrs 25 mins

Servings: 8

Yield: 8 servings

Ingredients

6 skinless, boneless chicken breast halves

3 (14.5 ounce) cans diced tomatoes

1 (16 ounce) jar green salsa

1 (15 ounce) can black beans, rinsed and drained

1 (15 ounce) can pinto beans, drained and rinsed

1 (15.25 ounce) can whole kernel corn, drained

1 (1.25 ounce) package taco seasoning

1 tablespoon chopped fresh cilantro

2 teaspoons ground red chile pepper, or to taste

1 teaspoon ground cumin

½ cup cream cheese, softened

Directions

Instructions

Step 1

Place the chicken breasts into the bottom of a slow cooker, and pour tomatoes, green salsa, black beans, pinto beans, and corn over the chicken. Sprinkle taco seasoning, cilantro, ground red chile, and cumin over the mixture, and stir to combine. Cover the cooker, set on Low, and cook until chicken is very tender and the mixture has thickened, 8 to 10 hours.

Step 2

For soup, leave all liquid in the cooker; for a thicker stew, remove some liquid if desired. Mix 1 or 2 tablespoons of liquid with cream cheese in a bowl, stir until smooth, and mix the cream cheese into the cooker to make a creamy sauce. Continue to cook for 15 minutes, then serve.

Cook's Note

You can certainly use this recipe as a base for incredible creamy tortilla soup too. Using one of those pre-roasted chickens or turkeys from your local grocery, shred and place in the bottom of the cooker instead of chicken breasts.

Nutrition Facts

Per Serving:

331 calories; protein 26g; carbohydrates 37g; fat 7.9g; cholesterol 61.6mg; sodium 1301.8mg.

Colleen's Slow Cooker Jambalaya

Recipe Summary

prep: 20 mins

cook: 8 hrs

total: 8 hrs 20 mins

Servings: 12

Yield: 12 servings

Ingredients

1 pound skinless, boneless chicken breast halves - cut into 1 inch cubes

1 pound andouille sausage, sliced

1 (28 ounce) can diced tomatoes with juice

1 large onion, chopped

1 large green bell pepper, chopped

1 cup chopped celery

1 cup chicken broth

2 teaspoons dried oregano

2 teaspoons dried parsley

2 teaspoons Cajun seasoning

1 teaspoon cayenne pepper

½ teaspoon dried thyme

1 pound frozen cooked shrimp without tails

Directions

Instructions

Step 1

In a slow cooker, mix the chicken, sausage, tomatoes with juice, onion, green bell pepper, celery, and broth. Season with oregano, parsley, Cajun seasoning, cayenne pepper, and thyme.

Step 2

Cover, and cook 7 to 8 hours on Low, or 3 to 4 hours on High. Stir in the shrimp during the last 30 minutes of cook time.

Nutrition Facts

Per Serving:

235 calories; protein 20.2g; carbohydrates 6.1g; fat 13.6g; cholesterol 98.9mg; sodium 687.6mg.

Hearty Turkey Soup with Parsley Dumplings

Recipe Summary

Servings: 8

Yield: 8 serving

Ingredients

1 picked over turkey carcass

12 cups water

1 ½ cups chopped celery

5 carrots

1 yellow onion, cut into wedges

2 teaspoons salt

¾ teaspoon dried thyme

1 cube chicken bouillon

1 bay leaf

6 tablespoons all-purpose flour

½ cup milk

1 small rutabaga, cubed

½ teaspoon ground black pepper

1 ½ pounds cooked turkey, cubed

½ cup chopped fresh parsley

2 slices white bread, quartered

1 ¼ cups all-purpose flour

1 teaspoon baking powder

¼ teaspoon salt

½ cup milk

4 tablespoons butter, melted

Directions

Instructions

Step 1

Combine turkey carcass, water, 1 cup celery, 2 carrots, onion, 2 teaspoons salt, thyme, bouillon, and bay leaf in large 4 quart stockpot. Bring to boiling. Lower heat, and cover. Simmer for 1 1/2 hours. Strain stock, and discard solids. Skim off fat using ladle or fat separator. Pick meat off bones when cooled. Reserve meat.

Step 2

Combine 6 tablespoons flour and 1/2 cup milk in a jar with a tight fitting lid. Shake to combine. Pour stock into pot. Bring to simmering. Strain flour mixture through sieve into stock, stirring.

Step 3

Slice remaining 3 carrots. Add rutabaga, ground pepper, remaining 1/2 cup celery, and sliced carrots. Simmer 20 minutes, or until vegetables are tender.

Step 4

While the soup is simmering, prepare the dumplings. Combine parsley and bread in processor; whirl until medium size crumbs. Add 1 1/4 cups flour, baking powder, and salt; process just until combined. Add 1/2 cup milk and butter; process using on-off pulses just until blended.

Step 5

Drop mounded tablespoons of dumpling mixture into simmering soup. Place cover on pot. Cook for 12 minutes, or until dumplings are dry in center. Add turkey meat; cook 3 minutes, or until heated through.

Nutrition Facts

Per Serving:

404 calories; protein 29.9g; carbohydrates 32.2g; fat 16.7g; cholesterol 91.3mg; sodium 1067mg.

Vegan Mushroom Ceviche

Recipe Summary

prep: 25 mins

cook: 10 mins

additional: 20 mins

total: 55 mins

Servings: 6

Yield: 6 servings

Ingredients

3 tablespoons olive oil

2 cloves garlic, chopped

3 (8 ounce) packages fresh white mushrooms, chopped

salt to taste

6 tomatoes, chopped

2 carrots, grated

1 white onion, chopped

2 tablespoons chopped fresh cilantro

1 fresh serrano pepper, seeded and chopped

1 pickled jalapeno pepper, seeded and chopped

½ cup lime juice

½ cup tomato juice

½ cup ketchup

2 tablespoons pickled jalapeno pepper juice

2 avocados - peeled, pitted, and sliced

Directions

Instructions

Step 1

Heat olive oil in a large skillet over medium heat. Add garlic and cook for 10 seconds. Stir in mushrooms and season with salt; cook until soft, about 8 minutes. Remove from heat.

Step 2

Place mushrooms in a large bowl and add tomatoes, carrots, onion, cilantro, serrano pepper, and jalapeno pepper.

Step 3

Combine lime juice, tomato juice, ketchup, and pickle juice in a second bowl. Pour over mushroom mixture and let stand for 20 minutes. Serve garnished with avocado slices.

Nutrition Facts

Per Serving:

253 calories; protein 6.9g; carbohydrates 24.2g; fat 17.4g; sodium 389.5mg.

Easy Slow Cooker Chicken and Dumplings
Recipe Summary

prep: 20 mins

cook: 5 hrs

total: 5 hrs 20 mins

Servings: 8

Yield: 8 servings

Ingredients

¼ cup water, or as needed

1 teaspoon poultry seasoning

salt and ground black pepper to taste

4 skinless, boneless chicken breast halves

1 (10.75 ounce) can low-sodium chicken broth, divided

1 large onion, finely diced

3 carrots, chopped

4 stalks celery, chopped

2 tablespoons butter

1 (10.75 ounce) can reduced-fat condensed cream of celery soup (such as Campbell's®)

1 (10.75 ounce) can reduced-fat condensed cream of chicken soup (such as Campbell's® Healthy Request)

½ teaspoon dried rosemary

1 (10 ounce) package refrigerated biscuit dough, torn into pieces

Directions

Instructions

Step 1

Whisk water, poultry seasoning, salt, and black pepper together in a bowl; add chicken to bowl and turn to coat.

Step 2

Pour 1/2 of the chicken broth into a slow cooker; add chicken and poultry seasoning mixture. Layer onion, carrots, and celery, respectively, over chicken. Dot butter over vegetables; pour celery soup and chicken soup over vegetables and sprinkle rosemary on top.

Step 3

Cook on High for 3 1/2 to 4 1/2 hours. Remove chicken from slow cooker and shred with two forks; return chicken to slow cooker. Add biscuit dough pieces to chicken mixture. Cook on High for 1 1/2 hours.

Nutrition Facts

Per Serving:

270 calories; protein 16.1g; carbohydrates 27.3g; fat 10.6g; cholesterol 43.9mg; sodium 755.3mg.

Mediterranean Shrimp with Tomatoes and Feta

Recipe Summary

prep: 15 mins

cook: 30 mins

total: 45 mins

Servings: 6

Yield: 6 servings

Ingredients

  6 large tomatoes, sliced 1/8-inch thick

  6 cloves garlic, minced

  3 tablespoons olive oil

  ¾ teaspoon salt

¾ teaspoon ground black pepper

1 ½ pounds uncooked medium shrimp, peeled and deveined

2 tablespoons lemon juice

1 cup crumbled feta cheese

½ cup chopped fresh parsley

Directions

Instructions

Step 1

Preheat the oven to 450 degrees F (230 degrees C).

Step 2

Place tomatoes in the bottom of a 9x13-inch baking dish. Add garlic and olive oil and combine. Sprinkle with salt and pepper.

Step 3

Place on the top rack of the preheated oven and roast for 20 minutes.

Step 4

Remove the dish from the oven, leaving oven on. Stir in shrimp and lemon juice. Sprinkle with feta cheese.

Step 5

Return the dish to the oven and continue to cook until shrimp are bright pink on the outside and meat is opaque, 10 to 15 minutes. Sprinkle with parsley.

Nutrition Facts

Per Serving:

298 calories; protein 26.5g; carbohydrates 10.5g; fat 17.1g; cholesterol 210mg; sodium 970.4mg.

Barbeque Seitan and Black Bean Burritos

Recipe Summary

prep: 30 mins

cook: 40 mins

total: 1 hr 10 mins

Servings: 10

Yield: 10 burritos

Ingredients

3 tablespoons olive oil

1 small onion, chopped

5 green onions, chopped

2 cloves garlic, minced

2 habanero peppers, seeded and minced

1 red bell pepper, chopped

1 ½ (8 ounce) packages seitan

1 (15 ounce) can black beans, rinsed and drained

1 (16 ounce) can diced tomatoes

3 cups cooked white rice

3 tablespoons chopped fresh cilantro

1 (18 ounce) bottle barbecue sauce

10 (10 inch) flour tortillas

Directions

Instructions

Step 1

In a large saucepan (wok pans also work well) heat oil over medium-high and saute yellow onion, green onions, garlic, habanero, and bell pepper until onions become translucent. Add seitan and saute another 5 minutes. Add black beans and tomatoes. Heat through.

Step 2

In a medium size mixing bowl combine heated mixture with cooked rice, cilantro, and 1 cup barbecue sauce.

Step 3

Lay tortillas on flat surface. Spoon about 3/4 cup of filling onto each tortilla's center. Wrap tortilla so that mixture is captured on the inside.

Step 4

In a casserole dish pour barbecue sauce to coat the dish's bottom. Place burritos in dish and pour more barbecue sauce on top of them. Bake in a preheated 350 degrees F (175 degrees C) oven for 35 minutes.

Cook's Note:

Most flour tortillas are vegetarian or vegan, but some may contain lard. Check the label.

Nutrition Facts

Per Serving:

509 calories; protein 18.3g; carbohydrates 83.7g; fat 5.3g; sodium 1240mg.

Recipe Summary

prep: 30 mins

cook: 10 mins

additional: 2 hrs

total: 2 hrs 40 mins

Servings: 6

Yield: 6 servings

Ingredients

1 cup olive oil

¼ cup chopped fresh parsley

1 lemon, juiced

2 tablespoons hot pepper sauce

3 cloves garlic, minced

1 tablespoon tomato paste

2 teaspoons dried oregano

1 teaspoon salt

1 teaspoon ground black pepper

2 pounds large shrimp, peeled and deveined with tails attached

skewers

Directions

Instructions

Step 1

In a mixing bowl, mix together olive oil, parsley, lemon juice, hot sauce, garlic, tomato paste, oregano, salt, and black pepper. Reserve a small amount for basting later. Pour remaining marinade into a large resealable plastic bag with shrimp. Seal, and marinate in the refrigerator for 2 hours.

Step 2

Preheat grill for medium-low heat. Thread shrimp onto skewers, piercing once near the tail and once near the head. Discard marinade.

Step 3

Lightly oil grill grate. Cook shrimp for 5 minutes per side, or until opaque, basting frequently with reserved marinade.

Note

The nutrition data for this recipe includes information for the full amount of the marinade ingredients. Depending on marinating time, ingredients, cooking method, etc., the actual amount of the marinade consumed will vary.

Nutrition Facts

Per Serving:

447 calories; protein 25.3g; carbohydrates 3.7g; fat 37.5g; cholesterol 230.4mg; sodium 800mg.

Creamy Mushroom Meatloaf

Recipe Summary

prep: 15 mins

cook: 2 hrs

total: 2 hrs 15 mins

Servings: 8

Yield: 8 servings

Ingredients

¼ cup butter

2 cups shiitake mushrooms, sliced

1 pinch salt

1 sprig fresh rosemary, chopped

3 tablespoons all-purpose flour

2 ½ cups beef broth

salt and pepper to taste

½ cup heavy cream

1 (2 1/2 pound) uncooked prepared beef, veal and pork meatloaf

Directions

Instructions

Step 1

Preheat the oven to 325 degrees F (165 degrees C).

Step 2

Melt butter in an oven-safe skillet over medium-high heat. Stir in mushrooms and a pinch of salt; cook and stir until mushrooms begin to brown, about 5 minutes.

Step 3

Stir in fresh rosemary. Add flour and stir to coat the mushrooms; cook and stir for about 3 minutes.

Step 4

Whisk in beef broth, 1/2 cup at a time, whisking constantly to prevent lumps.

Step 5

Turn heat to high and bring the sauce to a simmer. Simmer a few minutes until sauce starts to thicken. Season with salt and pepper to taste.

Step 6

Remove from heat and stir in heavy cream.

Step 7

Slide prepared meatloaf into the sauce. Spoon sauce over the top of the meatloaf.

Step 8

Bake in the preheated oven until no longer pink in the center, about 1 1/2 hours. An instant-read thermometer inserted into the center should read at least 160 degrees F (70 degrees C).

Step 9

Remove pan from the oven and gently remove meatloaf to a serving platter.

Step 10

Skim off any extra fat from the surface of the sauce.

Step 11

Bring the sauce to a boil over medium-high heat to reduce until thick, about 5 minutes.

Cook's Notes:

Use any recipe you like for the meatloaf. Nutritional information is for a 2 1/2 pound beef, veal and pork meatloaf. Try this recipe for Classic Meatloaf, which calls for ground chuck. Or use 1.5 pounds ground beef, 1 pound ground pork.

Using cold beef broth keeps the flour from forming lumps.

Nutrition Facts

Per Serving:

324 calories; protein 27.9g; carbohydrates 13.6g; fat 16.5g; cholesterol 138.6mg; sodium 501.1mg.

Mediterranean Quinoa Salad

Recipe Summary

prep: 15 mins

cook: 20 mins

total: 35 mins

Servings: 8

Yield: 4 cups

Ingredients

2 cups water

2 cubes chicken bouillon

1 clove garlic, smashed

1 cup uncooked quinoa

2 large cooked chicken breasts - cut into bite size pieces

1 large red onion, diced

1 large green bell pepper, diced

½ cup chopped kalamata olives

½ cup crumbled feta cheese

¼ cup chopped fresh parsley

¼ cup chopped fresh chives

½ teaspoon salt

⅔ cup fresh lemon juice

1 tablespoon balsamic vinegar

¼ cup olive oil

Directions

Instructions

Step 1

Bring the water, bouillon cubes, and garlic to a boil in a saucepan. Stir in the quinoa, reduce heat to medium-low, cover, and simmer until the quinoa is tender and the water has been absorbed, 15 to 20 minutes. Discard the garlic clove and scrape the quinoa into a large bowl.

Step 2

Gently stir the chicken, onion, bell pepper, olives, feta cheese, parsley, chives, and salt into the quinoa. Drizzle with the lemon juice, balsamic vinegar, and olive oil. Stir until evenly mixed. Serve warm or refrigerate and serve cold.

Nutrition Facts

Per Serving:

278 calories; protein 18.4g; carbohydrates 20.1g; fat 13.9g; cholesterol 44.6mg; sodium 713.1mg.

Tomato-Cream Sauce for Pasta

Recipe Summary

prep: 5 mins

cook: 15 mins

total: 20 mins

Servings: 5

Yield: 5 servings

Ingredients

2 tablespoons olive oil

1 onion, diced

1 clove garlic, minced

1 (14.5 ounce) can Italian-style diced tomatoes, undrained

1 tablespoon dried basil leaves

¾ teaspoon white sugar

¼ teaspoon dried oregano

¼ teaspoon salt

⅛ teaspoon ground black pepper

½ cup heavy cream

1 tablespoon butter

Directions

Instructions

Step 1

In a saucepan, saute onion and garlic in olive oil over medium heat. Make sure it doesn't burn. Add tomatoes, basil, sugar, oregano, salt and pepper. Bring to boil and continue to boil 5 minutes or until most of the liquid evaporates. Remove from heat; stir in whipping cream and butter. Reduce heat and simmer 5 more minutes.

Nutrition Facts

Per Serving:

182 calories; protein 1.7g; carbohydrates 6.7g; fat 16.6g; cholesterol 38.7mg; sodium 270.3mg.

Grill Master Chicken Wings

Recipe Summary

prep: 10 mins

cook: 20 mins

total: 30 mins

Servings: 10

Yield: 10 servings

Ingredients

Wings:

½ cup soy sauce

½ cup Italian-style salad dressing

3 pounds chicken wings, cut apart at joints, wing tips discarded

Sauce:

¼ cup butter

1 teaspoon soy sauce

¼ cup hot pepper sauce (such as Frank's RedHot®), or to taste

Directions

Instructions

Step 1

Combine 1/2 cup soy sauce, Italian dressing, and chicken wings in a large, zip-top bag. Close bag and refrigerate 4 hours to overnight.

Step 2

Preheat an outdoor grill for medium heat. In a small saucepan, melt the butter. Stir in the 1 teaspoon soy sauce and the hot pepper sauce. Turn off heat and reserve.

Step 3

Remove the chicken wings from the marinade and pat dry. Cook the wings on the preheated grill, turning occasionally, until the chicken is well browned and no longer pink, 25 to 30 minutes.

Step 4

Place grilled wings in a large bowl. Pour butter sauce over wings; toss to mix well.

Editor's Note

The nutrition data for this recipe includes the full amount of the marinade ingredients. The actual amount of the marinade consumed will vary.

Nutrition Facts

Per Serving:

181 calories; protein 10.1g; carbohydrates 2.3g; fat 14.6g; cholesterol 40.8mg; sodium 1154.1mg.

Cobb Salad
Recipe Summary

prep: 20 mins

cook: 30 mins

total: 50 mins

Servings: 6

Yield: 6 servings

Ingredients

6 slices bacon

3 eggs

1 head iceberg lettuce, shredded

3 cups chopped, cooked chicken meat

2 tomatoes, seeded and chopped

¾ cup blue cheese, crumbled

1 avocado - peeled, pitted and diced

3 green onions, chopped

1 (8 ounce) bottle Ranch-style salad dressing

Directions

Instructions

Step 1

Place eggs in a saucepan and cover completely with cold water. Bring water to a boil. Cover, remove from heat, and let eggs stand in hot water for 10 to 12 minutes. Remove from hot water, cool, peel and chop.

Step 2

Place bacon in a large, deep skillet. Cook over medium high heat until evenly brown. Drain, crumble and set aside.

Step 3

Divide shredded lettuce among individual plates.

Step 4

Evenly divide and arrange chicken, eggs, tomatoes, blue cheese, bacon, avocado and green onions in a row on top of the lettuce.

Step 5

Drizzle with your favorite dressing and enjoy.

Nutrition Facts

Per Serving:

525 calories; protein 31.7g; carbohydrates 10.2g; fat 39.9g; cholesterol 179.1mg; sodium 915.2mg.

www.ingramcontent.com/pod-product-compliance
Lightning Source LLC
Chambersburg PA
CBHW052126150726
48002CB00006B/2501